Your Breath, Your Life.

A Simple Guide to Pranayama and Breathwork

Dermot Ryan B.A.

OM Sahana Vavatu

Sahanau Bhunaktu

Saha Viryam Karavavahai

Tejasvi Navaditamastu

Ma Vidvishavahai

OM Shantih, Shantih, Shantih

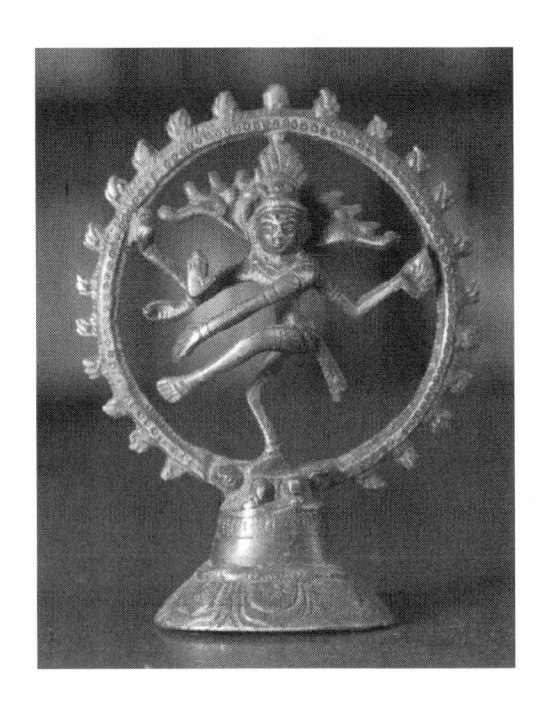

Text© Dermot Ryan 2020

Photography© Dermot Ryan 20

The information in this book has been compiled by way of general guidance in relation to the specific subject addressed. It is not a substitute and not to be relied on for medical, healthcare, pharmaceutical or other professional advice on specific circumstances and in specific locations. If you have any concerns about doing any of the breating exercises in the book, please consult with your doctor or physician. **For individuals with heart/lung issues, hypertension and pregnancy, the exercises contained in this book should only be practiced under the supervision of a qualified teacher**

No part of this publication may be reproduced, by any means, without the prior written permission of the author.

Requests for permission should be sent to: dryanyoga@gmail.com

To find out more about the author, please visit:
http://www.dermotryanyoga.com

The right of Dermot Ryan to be identified as author of this work has been asserted by him in accordance with the Copyright and Related Rights Act 2000 (Ireland)

CONTENTS

1. Introduction 1
2. And so, the story begins 4
3. What is Pranayama? What is Breathwork? 9
4. What is Prana? 12
5. The Basic Science Bit 16
6. The Art of Shutting your Mouth 21
7. Practice, Practice, and then, PRACTICE 24
8. Stretch Your Body 27
9. Just Sit Down! 29
10. What will I do with my Hands? 32
11. Learn to Breath (Three Part Breathing – Dirga) 35
12. Ujjayi Breath – Breath of Victory 40
13. Samma Vritti…Square Breathing 42
14. Kapalabhati (Shining Skull) 46
15. Bhastrika – The Bellows Breath 50
17. Nadi Shodhana – Alternate Nostril Breathing 56
18. Anuloma Viloma – A.N.B. w/Breath Retention 60
19. Surya and Chandra Bheda – The Sun, Moon 63
20. Sitali and Sitkari Pranayama – Cooling/Hissing Breath 66
21. Just say NO!..The joys of Nitric Oxide 68
22. Black Bee Breath – Brahmari 72
23. Other Breathing Methods 75
24. Relax like a Corpse – Play Dead 80
25. Conclusion 83
Dermot Ryan 85

1. Introduction

I was introduced to the benefits of proper breathing, Pranayama and Breathwork at a late stage in my life. I was 51 when I first sat down, closed my mouth, and took a deep long breath down into my belly. Since then I have taught hundreds of students these techniques during my Yoga classes and through workshops I run here in Ireland and online.

Recently, the Breath has become a very popular topic. There has been a myriad of articles in health magazines and weekend supplements. The "breath" is on an upward trend in the public mind. While many of the articles and even books tell us of the importance of breathing properly, they seem to skirt around giving a method for starting a breathwork/pranayama practice and how to build one.

So, instead of saying," I could do that", I put my knowledge garnered over the years down on paper and wrote a book. I based it on my experience, learning from recognised masters in India along with my study and practice. It is also a reflection of my own workshops and classes.

It should be noted that included in the title of this book is the word "simple". This is a simple guide to Pranayama and Breathwork. I have purposefully avoided biological diagrams, charts, and artists impression of energy moving through the body. This book is, as they say in India, for the Householder. I have tried to make the subject as accessible as possible to the widest range of people and so promote this health benefit to as many people as possible. This book will give you the foundation for a sustainable healthy practice and if you want to advance to the higher levels, there are other books for that, and caves and Ashrams to visit too.

My YouTube Channel has a guide to all the practices described in this book. If you need help, please contact me with any queries you may have, via my Website, Facebook, or Instagram.

Before signing off and letting you begin your journey, I need to give thanks and bow to those who assisted and supported me on this journey. My teachers, Sunil Ramachandran, Bhooma Chaitanya, Swami Govindananda. The great Karma Yogi, Gopalkrishna Baliga of Udupi, and Sivananda Yoga Vidya Peetham (Kerala).

My loyal Yoga students who have travelled this path with me, even when I dragged them to India (!). I thank you all.

Last, my undying thanks to my wife Rosemarie, who gave me the freedom to take this journey. She was my biggest supporter and fan, helped me fulfil my dream, while sacrificing the "normal" path in life. Love you to the Moon and Back...

Om Tat Sat

Dermot

Galway, Ireland.

September 2020

2. And so, the story begins

It was March 2016 and I had travelled from Trivandrum, southern Kerala, India, north, to a dusty village outside Kollam. The three-hour road trip by taxi, with intermittent air conditioning, had been the usual Keralan colourful experience: unrelenting heat, noisy, elephants, monkeys, and colourful roadside markets, all covered in dust. This was not new to me. I had been to India many times but had not lost my sense of wonder, a pre-requisite for all travel in this part of our world. I should have asked the taxi driver to stop for a chai and a smoke on the way north, but we had chatted all the way, the time had flown by and now we had arrived at what would be my home for the next 35 days.

I paid my driver, stood at the gates of the Panmana Ashram and looked at this Soviet Style 4 storey block with a huge red tiled roof, a Hindu Temple in the forecourt, surrounded by coconut palms, and thought, this is very far from home! I was here to do my first Yoga Teacher Training and I had everything I needed with me, all my loose fitting clothes, a Yoga Mat, and being a 40 year smoking veteran, 400 Duty Free Cigarettes packed neatly in my small bag.. What could possibly go wrong? I should have stopped on the way up here! I was dying for a cigarette!

The first thing a veteran smoker does when arriving anywhere is to scan the area for smoking zones. This is a split-second mental operation; scan for peaceful place out of view, lodge in mind, and return later for quiet smoke...Easy...never failed. As I walked into the courtyard, past the Temple and into the large hall and reception area, I had still not found a place, which was a little disconcerting. There were lots of people, which always is a surprise in rural India, lots of windows, balconies and walkways overlooking every square inch of the property. I would have to try a little harder. Checking into my room, I saw the dreaded grills high on the walls between the rooms. No chance of smoking here! A slight panic emerges. I unpack, placing my 400 cigarettes at the back of my wardrobe, change my cloths, pick up my Yoga Mat and climb the stairs to the roof and begin the first Yoga class of my training.

I had been introduced to Yoga a few years earlier on a visit to Kerala and had begun a daily practice 2.5 years earlier and this Teacher Training was the next step on this Yoga journey. I still smoked 20 cigarettes a day, still had a persistent smokers' cough and could not laugh deeply without coughing up phlegm. I loved smoking and had no intention of quitting! I loved the quote attributed to B.K.S. Iyengar, "Smoking won't affect your Yoga, but Yoga may affect your smoking"

Back to my first class of this training. It was really my first introduction to Pranayama Breathing Techniques. My Yoga was all self-practice, so Pranayama was not part of what I did. I had seen it, but it was difficult to integrate these practices without a proper teacher, and now I had one. We moved slowly through the introduction with each practice being explained slowly and precisely. Our teacher BhoomaJi stressed the importance of slow progress as he introduced each new practice. As we finished this class, I felt more relaxed than usual and would even say slightly, euphoric.

I needed a cigarette!

Cold shower, dinner and bed came in quick succession and no opportunity to be alone and smoke. Up at 6 a.m. for nasal cleansing class and then more Pranayama and Yoga. This is when everything felt different. After our breathing practice, my Yoga practice felt different. I was breathing deeper and longer. I was releasing tension and feeling a new energy moving through my body. What was most surprising was, the rattle in my chest was gone. I mean completely gone! I hadn't coughed, spluttered or spat when I got up that morning, as I had done for many years. In just 12 hours and two Pranayama sessions, my lungs felt renewed and clear of that fluffy and congested feeling which I had grown used to. There was no rattle, no blocked feeling, just a freedom in my breathing that was long lost to me…The feeling of panic that had been in my body had subsided. Maybe I had received my first lesson in non-attachment….

I never smoked again…After two months in India, I brought 400 cigarettes home to Ireland and they eventually mysteriously disappeared. I have suspects!

That was the beginning of my relationship with Pranayama, the power of our breath to heal and its' myriad of benefits. I have been an acolyte ever since, and through this book, I hope you will gain the knowledge of this ancient practice that will help you lead a long, and healthier life.

3. What is Pranayama? What is Breathwork?

I generally start my Breathwork and Pranayama Workshops with a question and a sales pitch.

Are you willing to give a little time each day to a practice that will and is proven to make your skin shine, reduce wrinkles and ageing? It does not involve taking a tablet, but it does involve ingesting a colourless, invisible naturally occurring substance. You would be intrigued. Furthermore, it can help with digestion and digestive issues. It can increase energy levels. It can help concentration and brain power. It can help you sleep longer and deeper. It can cure migraine and lower back pain. It can help you lose weight. It will help you live longer and more importantly; it will help you live a longer healthier life. It will reduce the chances that you will suffer from depression and overall, because of all these benefits, it will give you a better chance of being happier. Generally, the participants want at least one of these things and usually and not surprisingly they want them all. As the whole room is reaching for their cheque books and credit cards,

I explain that this wonder cure is available to them by just learning how to breathe properly and by taking a little time each day to practice...

For hundreds, if not thousands of years, these practices were kept secret by small groups of practitioners and Yogis on the Indian sub-continent. Even the ancient Yoga texts say that these practices must be kept secret and that only those properly initiated by a Guru should practice. Of course, over the years there has been scepticism about these esoteric practices in the West but with new studies at major Universities these methods have now been proved to be of unprecedented benefit to our health and wellbeing. Not only are the myriad of benefits, physical, but because the breath has such an effect on the mind, the mental health benefits are astounding. In the ancient text, the Hatha Yoga Pradipika, the author tells us that, like training wild animals, the air in the body can be gradually brought under control using the correct methods. Once the air is controlled, the mind is controlled and if a person can control the mind, then he controls the air. Not only were the Indian Yogis discovering the power of the breath, but

Hippocrates, the father of medicine had a similar view to power of proper breathing. In his view, unregulated breathing was the cause of disease and all other things are secondary and subordinate causes. Taking both ideas together, we arrive at the basic principle of Pranayama and Breathwork.

And the LORD God formed man of the dust of the ground and breathed into his nostrils the breath of life; and man became a living soul. Genesis 2:7

4. What is Prana?

According to Swami Sivananda, "Prana is the sum total of all the energy in the Universe". Everything that moves in the Universe is a manifestation of Prana. Life attracts Prana to itself, stores it, and transforms it both internally and externally. Prana exists in everything but not in any one thing. Air, water, food, sunlight all transport Prana. It is what really nourishes us, and without it, there is no life. Vitality is no more than a subtle form of Prana. The science of controlling Prana is called Pranayama...

It is generally explained by comparing it to electricity in our daily lives. We can look at all the appliances we use every day without ever thinking about what makes them work. The unseen force that flows through each part of a machine. It only becomes an issue with a power outage. In fact, electricity itself is a manifestation of Prana.

By breathing properly and using different techniques, we try to control this force in our bodies. We try to "curb" and "master" it. The Sanskrit for this is "ayama", so to curb and master the breath is called Pranayama. The breath is the vehicle that transports Prana into our bodies.

This mastery is what leads Yogis to take control of all parts of their internal and external bodies. We have all seen the heart control displays under laboratory conditions performed by Eastern Monks and Yogis. Even though they violate physiological laws during these prolonged exercises of organ control, they enjoy robust health and wellbeing.

The idea and concept of Prana can be a little incomprehensible and confusing to us in the western world. Labelling it "life-force" or "energy" gives us only a glimpse of its real power and omnipresence. Our awareness of its presence is heightened by Pranayama practice, inner silence, and mindful actions.

Prana moves throughout our bodies. This movement of Prana is called Prana Vayu or "wind" and is broken up into 5 separate Vayus, covering the whole body.

They are:

1. **Udana Vayu**: This is an upward and outward movement of energy. It governs inspiration

and enthusiasm and the Udana moves the Prana upwards towards the throat and face during inhalation. Retaining the breath after inhalation affects Udana Vayu in this area, holding it steadily and nourishing this area of the body.

2. **Prana Vayu**: This is the inward and upward movement of energy. It governs sensory experience, mental experiences, eating, drinking and our inhalation. It increases energy and vitality. This Vayu is controlled by the inhalation and controls the prana as it rises from the chest.

3. **Samana Vayu**: This is the inward-spiralling movement of energy, also known as the Vayu of Assimilation. This Vayu governs the assimilation of food and oxygen into our bodies. Samans spirals this prana around our navel centre and is affected but steady and balanced inhalation and exhalation.

4. **Apana Vayu**: This is the downward and outward movement of energy. This Vayu governs the elimination of waste from the body. It also governs exhalation, childbirth, and the removal of negative emotional

experiences. Apana Vayu is affected by our exhalations during Pranayama.

5. **Vyana Vayu**: This is the circulating and expanding movement of energy. This Vayu governs nutrients in the blood and bodily fluid. It also governs our engagement with the world outside of ourselves, our thoughts, and emotions. This Vayu spirals outward from the centre of our bodies and moves out into the world beyond. Vyana Vayu is affected by controlling the capacity of both the inhalation and the exhalation.

5. The Basic Science Bit….

We come into this world with an **Inhale** and we leave this world with an **Exhale**. In between we take between 21,000 and 23,000 breaths per day. The Yoga Masters of India believe that when we are born, we are given a certain amount of breaths to use while in this world. Each breath must be used carefully to extend our lives for as long as possible, to burn off as much karma as possible, and be as healthy as possible for the whole of our lives.

Over thousands of years they have developed unique breathing exercises that help with the ideal of a long, healthy life. Proper Breathing is a very large part of Yoga Practice and is the 4th limb in the 8 Limbs of Yoga, known as Pranayama…A breathing practice has to be mastered before progressing to any form of mindfulness or meditation, finally leading to Enlightenment.

We are all aware of sayings that relate to our breath…"it takes my breath away" and even when a child is very upset, we encourage them to take "a deep breath" and to calm down. How our body really works is hard wired into our DNA. When it comes to our own health and wellbeing, we seem to ignore these inbuilt signals and continue doing the incorrect things.

Our nervous system is split into two separate areas...Our Sympathetic Nervous System (SNS) and our Parasympathetic Nervous System (PSNS). Our SNS is our in-built survival when in danger mechanism, our "Fight of Flight" reaction. Our PSNS is our "Rest and Digest" mechanism, which does what it says on the tin...we rest and digest...There are 8 areas in our body that relate to or Fight or Flight mechanism while there are 4 that relate to our Rest and Digest mechanism. Over the millennia our Fight or Flight reaction has been very important...If a lion or a tiger is chasing you and you go into rest and digest mode...then you would be known as "dinner". The fact that our ancestors survived, and we are here today is testament to the proper functioning and high performance of the Sympathetic Nervous System.

The difference between you and your ancestors is that, in this information age, we are "always on", digitally obsessed and in general our world is escape based. We are being bombarded by so many different types of media, pictures, images and information, all day, every day. When I use the term, "always on", I mean that we are living our lives in our SNS world and are ever ready for "Fight or Flight". We are on edge, anxious, nervous, and so on, just waiting for that TIGER, all the time. This is not news to us. This is obvious. We all know how this is affecting our health, our lives and most importantly, our relationships with others.

So, if your SNS is always on, that means that your PSNS is redundant, and always "off". This means, we never REST and we never DIGEST. With any muscle or system in the body, you "use it or lose it". If you have ever broken a bone and been in a cast for 4/6 weeks, you know that when the cast is removed, the muscles have degenerated massively and that it takes a long time to get them back to where they were, lots of physio etc. So, let us imagine not using your PSNS for years, never Resting and Digesting, always being in Fight or Flight mode. What has degenerated and what have we lost?

"I'm always exhausted, but I can't sleep, I can't slow down, sometimes I am on the verge of tears for no reason, I'm overwhelmed, I always have heart burn, my lower back is killing me, my neck is stiff, if I could just get someone to massage my shoulders, I'm on a diet and I can't lose weight".

These are the familiar statements that I regularly hear when teaching. One, or some of them resonate with many, if not most people. They are just a few examples of what we have lost. If you are feeling like this, what message are you giving to your family, partners work colleagues? How are these statements, even one of them effecting your relationships? How much "emotional medication" are you taking to relieve these symptoms? Having a glass of wine to take the edge off is probably the emotional and physical pain reliever of choice these days.

How do we tap into this "Rest and Digest" magic potion, and turn on our PSNS? I mentioned earlier there are 4 areas of out body that are connected to our PSNS as against 8 for our SNS...These 4 areas are our Eyes, Our Jaw Bones, Our Smile, and our Gut. Our gut is connected to our heart, lungs, digestive system and so on...and all of this is controlled by what we call, The Vagus Nerve, the

Latin for wanderer, appropriately called because it wanders all over your upper body. To turn it on and start using it, get the myriad of benefits from it, all you must do is Breathe. You need to Breath, but not like you breathe now. You need to really breath, re-learn something you do over 21,000 times per day, and then, slowly develop a daily practice. Even if this practice is only for 5/10 minutes per day, it is your gateway to reaping all the benefits of these ancient practices.

"The Breath opens the window into ourselves, making the unconscious, conscious" – Adrian Cox, Breath Yoga

6. The Art of Shutting your Mouth

Is a simple thing like letting air in and out of your mouth and down into your lungs, creating a you that is no longer functioning to your full health potential? The answer is, a resounding, Yes. Read any writings by renowned Buteko breathing specialist, Patrick McKeown or even the short experiment by James Nestor in his recent book, "Breath".

Why are these habits bad for your health? Why do you need to learn to do something that you have been doing since birth and that you do without thinking every minute of every day? You started your life as the perfect breather and despite what we think, when babies are not crying, they have their mouths shut and are breathing in and out through their nostrils. As we grow up, we unlearn this and slowly our heavy jaw begins to drop. We start breathing mostly through or mouths. We have become the only animals on the planet that mouth breath.

If we are not doing this, we are, what is termed "gymnastic" breathing. We are expanding our chest when inhaling and contracting our chest when exhaling. We pull our abdomen in when we inhale and relax our abdomen when we exhale.

A further habit we tend to develop is vertical breathing. This is the habit of letting our shoulders rise on an inhale and drop down when exhaling.

These three most common breathing habits are having a detrimental effect on our health and I could go as far as to say, killing us. It is hard to believe that breathing can kill you. Let me be a little less dramatic. Breathing incorrectly is "slowly" killing you. It is also increasing your dental bills. It is stopping you controlling your weight. It is giving you asthma and reducing your lung capacity. It is giving you lower back pain. It is increasing damaging issues with your neck and shoulders. It is increasing your risk of having cardiac and lung problems. It is affecting your ability to control your weight. It is giving you sleepless nights and probably giving your partner and family sleepless nights too. Your snoring and sleep apnea are a direct result of a mouth breathing habit. It is damaging your health in these and many other ways. The art of un-learning these bad breathing habits is one of the most easily accessible health remedies available. To speed up the process and benefit from nasal breathing while sleeping, taping the mouth shut can produce great benefits.

The biggest threat to your overall health and wellbeing is mouth breathing. The three words**,** **Shut Your Mouth**, will save you endless problems. Get into the habit of repeating this mantra to yourself throughout your day. It will help you unlearn bad habits. It will be your first guide on the road of new breathing techniques.

7. Practice, Practice, and then, PRACTICE

In late 2013, I asked my Yoga teacher Sunil, what was the best time of day to practice mediation. The answer made me laugh, "one and a half hours before dawn", he said. I was to learn later that the mind is inherently still at that time, enabling one to achieve a deeper meditative state. I was also to learn that it is the best time to practice Breathwork and Pranayama.

It is late February 2018, it is 430am, I am sitting cross-legged on the rooftop of a 4-storey building in Northern Kerala. I am attending an advanced teacher training here for one month. Getting up at 4am is the new "normal". It is no laughing matter! We have completed our Kriya cleansing, washing our nasal passages out with warm salted water and pulling a catheter through our nose, down into our throats and out our mouths. The sound of choking and spitting fills the early morning air. We then climb the stairs to the rooftop and complete rounds of Sun Salutations and then settle down. The air is cool and the 25 of us are wrapped in our shawls and blankets in a large semi-circle. Our teacher Swami Govindananda begins the session with a health warning, as he does every day before we begin our Pranayama practice. Do not push your body, do not put your body under any stress, do not become breathless. Stay with the limits of your bodies' abilities. Listen to your body, intensely. It will last one and a half hours. We go through each exercise, guided slowly and precisely. We drift in and out of meditative states with a voice guiding us to breathe deeply, to hold our breath in our bodies, to hold our breath outside of our bodies, to feel the energy of the breath in the very core of our bodies. The Sanskrit word **Sukha** probably describes the world that we enter each morning during this long practice – An authentic and lasting state of happiness. We finish every session with the Black Bee Pranayama (Brahmarhi)...humming and vibrating our sinuses while we inhale and exhale, creating Nitric Oxide in our nasal passage, inhaling it deep into our lungs, sterilising the air, causing the blood vessels to widen and lowering our blood pressure. At 6am, we feel ready to face the long day ahead. We fill the four hours before breakfast with a meditation walk, a cup of oat tea, chanting, a philosophy class and of course a Yoga class. After over thirty days of this continuous practice, a new awareness of the power of the breath is achieved.

As this intense practice is not practical in a normal life, it is important to see how to structure a practice, which suits your lifestyle. As in a meditation practice, it is important to try and practice at the same time and in the same place. The optimum benefit is achieved by daily practice. Take some time before and after to relax the body and mind. Do not try to do too much to begin, and slowly develop a habit.

The 21/90 Rule states that it takes 21 days to make a habit and 90 days to make it a permanent lifestyle change. Commit to your goal for 21 days and it will become a habit. Commit to your goal for 90 days and it will become a part of your lifestyle.

8.Stretch Your Body

There are eight limbs of Yoga and the fourth is Pranayama/Breathwork. The third limb is Postures/Asanas. These stages in a practice are not random and each stage gently eases the practitioner into the iteration of a complete practice. Taking this into account, it can be of great benefit to do some easy body stretches before focussing on the practice of breathing. We hold tension in our bodies, whether physical, emotional, or karmic. If we mentally scan our bodies, we can get a feel for places where these tensions are lodged. I always tell my students that the first place to check is the jaw and then move slowly around the body from there, mentally releasing tension as they move through the body, right down to the toes. Whether sitting, lying down, or standing, move your body into positions that are not usual for you. There is no need for a standard set of motions or poses for this practice. Maybe bend forward and try to touch your toes. Swing your arms slowly around your body. Lift your arms above your head. Look over your shoulders. Do whatever you feel your body needs and breath slowly and as deeply as you can. Stretch your exhalations out into the universe and let it carry the tension away. Bend your back, lean to the left and the right. Do what feels right for you and let this become a daily routine just for you. Make these movements your own personal gateway into a Breathing practice.

9.Just Sit Down!

We spend our lives breathing in lots of different positions. As you become more aware of "how to" breath and its' benefits you will find that the awareness of your breath becomes more apparent in your daily life. If we want to focus on our breath, develop a practice and explore various techniques, then seated positions are best for this. The most important aspect of any seated position is that your spine is straight and that you are comfortable and relaxed.

Because of our modern lifestyle, daily and hourly use of devices and computers, we are slumping forward more and more. Our "gait" or posture is becoming rounded, our upper back and shoulders slowly curving forward. If you think about this and maybe exaggerate this position, you will see how it effects your breathing. It restricts the movement of your diaphragm and the intake of breath into your lower lungs. You will find that are only using the upper part of your lungs. Even then, you are not using them to anywhere near optimum capacity.

Usually we are just taking short breaths and at too high a rate. We are over breathing.

To re-introduce proper functional breathing to our bodies, we need to reverse this creeping bad habit and re-assert a new posture into our daily lives. There are three ways to sit while practicing your breathing. No one is better than another, although the ancient texts say that certain cross-legged poses are preferable. For the western body, this is usually not comfortable or even possible.

If you decide to sit on the floor cross-legged and can do this for a period without discomfort of pain, then this is the classic position. Use cushions under the knees or buttocks if needed and try to tilt the hips forward. Push your navel out a little, straighten the spine. Try and maybe picture a string running through the top of your head, down through your spine and finishing at the base of the spine. Focus on this for a few breaths and you will feel a lengthening of the whole back. Keep your chin parallel to the floor. As you move through a breathing practice, you will find that the body will slump a little forward, but just repeat the straightening process after each exercise and eventually, it will happen less and less.

The other seated floor position is Thunderbolt Pose. In this position, you rest on your shins, with your buttocks on your heels, feet, and legs together. So, just get on your knees and relax back on to your heels. Repeat the process of straightening your spine and breath slowly and deeply to relax the body into the heels.

For most people, sitting on a chair is the optimum position for breathing exercises. It is preferable to use a hard chair and to sit forward, towards the front. Your spine should not be supported by the back of the chair. Both feet should be firmly and flat on the floor. As with the other two positions, go through the process of straightening the spine and rolling back the shoulders, so that the pressure on the lungs and abdomen is released.

When you are comfortable in any of these positions, then you are ready to begin your breathing practice. Each position is interchangeable, so it is perfectly fine to switch positions at any time, even during a session.

10. What will I do with my Hands?

We unconsciously use our hands to give signals to others and to our body and mind. It is a natural response to situations and emotions and we never even think about it. We are aware that certain cultures have different hand gestures to express feelings, emotions and even opinions, so it is not a new concept to any of us.

In Yoga we also use hand gestures and finger positions to give signals to our body. We tell it to move our internal energy (Prana) to certain areas or our body to repair, refresh and rejuvenate. You see these hand gestures in many Department Stores and Garden Centres where statues of the Buddha image are sold. Have you noticed that the Buddha has his hands in different positions while sitting cross-legged? These hand positions are called Mudras and they are a powerful aid to your Breathing practice. There are many books on Mudras, but for our practice, we will just focus on three. They are Chin Mudra, Jnana (Yana) Mudra and Dhyana (Diana) Mudra. Later we will introduce a fourth Mudra (Vishnu Mudra) as part of a specific breathing technique. Over a brief time, these Mudras will become second nature to you, and you can move between them at any time during your practice.

Chin/Jnana Mudra: Place the back of your hands on your thighs or knees, palms facing up towards the ceiling/sky. Connect the tip of your index finger to the tip of your thumb on both hands. A circle is formed between the two. Let you fingers relax and separate. This is Chin Mudra. This gesture represents the individual consciousness merging with the universal consciousness. This gesture invites us to be calm and helps generate a feeling of harmony with our environment and gives us a peaceful feeling. By turning your hands over and letting your palms face down, this becomes Jnana Mudra. While Chin Mudra lets us receive energy with open palms, Jnana Mudra helps us me be grounded. To control these two opposing energy gestures, it is also perfectly acceptable to have one hand in Chin Mudra and one hand in Jnana Mudra. Try out variations and see what feels good and is most beneficial for you. Your body has the answer. Listen to it and go slowly.

Dhyana Mudra: This is probably the most common Mudra that we are inadvertently aware of. The Buddha statue that you come across in various locations is generally sitting and his hands in Dhyana Mudra. The gesture is also used in Christian and European art also. Simply place your left hand in your lap, palm facing upwards. Then place the back of your right hand into your left hand, again with the palm facing up. Now connect the tips of both thumbs together. This is a direct signal to the mind that you want to go into meditation/relaxation mode. It generates a feeling of calm and most importantly for us, the mudra aides diaphragmatic breathing and leads to a still and focused mind. The unbroken flow of energy between the thumbs encourages better communication between the two hemispheres of the brain and leads to a more balance both in our body and mind.

11. Learn to Breath (Three Part Breathing – Dirga)

You have kept yourself alive for all these years, so you should really be an expert at breathing. Like everything else we do, we can fall into bad habits, so let us suspend all we think we know and begin.

Sit upright, out at the edge of your seat, so that your spine is not being supported. Try to picture your spine as a straight line from the chair all the way up to the base of your skull. Close your mouth! You only inhale and exhale through your nostrils….take a deep breath in …and exhale….and again…..and again….You will notice that when you do this, you slightly rise up when you inhale and move down when you exhale….Perfect? Well it is not perfect, at all.

Now, place your hands on your sides, your index fingers tucked slightly beneath your lowest rib. When you inhale, feel your elbows move away from your body. Now do this a few times….lovely….now keep your hands there, and we will do some more inhales and exhales, but when you inhale now, first, push your navel towards the wall in front of you, then let your elbows push out and then fill the upper part of your lungs and finally let the breath fill your throat. This is the three parts of correct breathing. If you like to add another layer, it might be nice to add another layer when beginning. So, four stages…belly, elbows, upper lungs, throat and then a nice long exhale. This may be very new to you and after many years of vertical breathing. It may feel strange and it is easy to slip back to habits shaped by many years of unconscious breathing habits. Stick with it and retrain your body and mind.

Now let us focus on the exhale. When you exhale, slowly let the air leave your throat, then your lungs and finally your belly. Pull your bellybutton/navel back in towards your spine, trying to push all the air out from the bottom of your lungs. Practice at a slow pace and do not put any stress into the action. Just do what is 100% comfortable and steady. Always try to make sure that your exhalation is longer than your inhalation…it is the exhalation that reduces your heart rate and your blood pressure…the optimum is that your exhalation is twice the length of your inhalation, but this comes with a lot of practice and concentration...This is correct breathing and it is probably a lot different from what you have been doing for all of your life. When I initially asked you to Inhale and Exhale, you were vertical breathing. Up and down, but you did not always do this. When you were born and for the first few years of your life, you breathed correctly, but then you became self-aware, you were told to stand tall, tuck in your tummy, have presence and this led you down the path of vertical or gymnastic breathing. This vertical motion places a lot of stress on your shoulders and neck. We spend a lot of our time on computers and other devices, leading to a myriad of neck and shoulder issues that are having an increasing negative impact on our health. If we repeat an incorrect motion 23,000 per day, every day, then the consequences can be easily identified.

Now that we have got to the stage of breathing correctly, I would like to explain how your breathing affects your brain. We all have a left side and a right-side brain. We use the left-hand side for administration, putting things in order, logic and so on. We use the right side of our brain for creativity, the arts etc. Our left and right brain are affected by the nostril that we inhale through. For the general population, the dominant or working nostril alternates from left to right and right to left every two to three hours. This can vary from person to person. Your dominant nostril is the nostril where the air flows freely. It is controlled by the central nervous system. For Indian Yogis who would have an intensive daily practice this would reduce to one to one and a half hours.

When you inhale through your left nostril, it oxygenates the right lobe of your brain and when you inhale through your right nostril it oxygenates the left lobe of your brain, so it is easy to see that if you are doing a maths exam and your left nostril is dominant and oxygenating the right side of your brain, this isn't going to be much help. You need to be breathing through your right nostril and oxygenating the left lobe of your brain. Generally, when you have difficulty focusing on the job at hand, it can be explained by which nostril is dominant and which lobe of the brain is being oxygenated.

It is possible to change the dominant nostril. For example, if you want to change the nostril dominance from left to right. Lie down and turn to the left side for ten minutes. This will help in shifting the active breathing to the right nostril. And vice versa.

It is also a good habit to check which nostril is dominant during your day and try to do tasks that suit the dominant nostril and brain. Try to be mindful of which nostril is dominant throughout your day.

12. Ujjayi Breath – Breath of Victory

I find that this very simple breathing technique really helps me to focus inwardly and shut out peripheral noise and sound in my immediate surroundings. It helps focus the mind on the breath and builds an awareness of the health of my breathing in the moment. Sometimes it sounds like cars on a wet road, the wind passing through trees and even Darth Vader, but it is a great tool to use at the beginning of a practice. It gives us the opportunity to judge the quality and smoothness of the breath. So, let us say, it is a preparatory exercise, a gateway to further practice. Using this technique with Samma Vritti (Square Breathing) is also recommended.

Simply put, we are constricting the flow of breath in our throat on both the inhale and the exhale. Of course, we are sitting in a comfortable position, with our spines straight and body relaxed. Our mouth is closed, and we are only breathing through our nostrils. Initially it may help to let your chin slightly drop towards your chest to get the feeling and sound of restricted breath, but once attained, lift the chin up, parallel to the floor. Even though the breath is slightly restricted, it should still flow softly and evenly on both the inhale and the exhale. The sound is the key to this, soft, even, effortless, subtle, and so on.

It can also be nice to play with the breath while using this technique. Inhale/Exhale for certain counts. Change the sound of the breath Use anything that stops the chattering of the mind and focusses you on the present moment. Try to breath longer and deeper than your normal breath, remembering the movements of proper breathing. Release physical and emotional tension when you exhale, let it all go. The jaw and the face are a good place to start. Eventually there will be an uninterrupted flow of breath and general relaxation.

I have seen it advised that people who are too introverted should not practice this breathing method.

13. Samma Vritti...Square Breathing

In Sanskrit, 'sama' = 'equal,' 'vritti' = 'flow,'. This practice teaches us to breath in four steps. This kind of breathing in English is called the Square Breathing or sometimes called Four Part Breathing. Our bodies are not used to this conscious breathing method as we generally breath subconsciously and we are not connected to the process. Square Breathing plays an important role, as it teaches you to be aware of the flow of the breath in the body and ultimately the flow of energy. We may be using and moving our diaphragms and abdomens incorrectly and so, this breathing method is used to train us to be more aware of the process. We become aware of the four distinct stages in the breathing process and this in turn bring us a little further along the path of improved breathing health and wellbeing.

The four steps are:
1. Inhalation
2. Retention after Inhalation
3. Exhalation

4. Retention after Exhalation. This can also be termed, holding the breath, or retaining the breath outside of the body.

To begin this practice, it is usual to start with using a count of 4 seconds, but as with all these practices, if this is a little stressful on your body, begin with a count 3. The duration of the breathing and holds can be increased through practice, but always remembering that each phase should be effortless and place no stress on the breath, always steady and comfortable. It is also recommended that if practitioners have difficulty with the four stages, then a three-stage alternative can be used to gain confidence and rhythm. This "triangle" method just skips the fourth stage, retention of the breath outside the body. So, we inhale, hold our breath and exhale, all for the same duration and progress slowly to the four-stage breathing when confidence and physical ability allow.

Benefits:
1. **Inhalation**
    - Improves lung capacity.
    - Wakes up the sluggish cells in the body.

- Encourages the right kind of breathing.
- Long and deep inhalation builds awareness.

2. **Retention**
   - The energy in the body stays calm.
   - The retained energy within the body stimulates the dull organs and the glands.
   - It distributes the energy equally within the entire body.
   - The retained energy can prepare the body for meditation.

3. **Exhalation**
   - Antioxidants are expelled from the body efficiently.
   - Helps to reduce stress and anxiety.
   - Keeps the diaphragm active.
   - Increases immunity.

4. **Retention after Exhalation**
   - The body becomes silent, as there is no movement of energy.
   - This silence calms the body and the mind physiologically and psychologically.

- Helps to control the state of mind and leads to deeper relaxation.

14.Kapalabhati (Shining Skull)

While generally regarded as a cleansing exercise, Kapalabhati is an ideal practice to prepare the body and lungs for an extended breathing practice. It is generally coupled with the Bellows Breath (Bhastrika) at the beginning of a practice. It is important to do at least one of these exercises at the beginning of your practice and it is preferable that both be done. Neither of these practices are recommended during pregnancy or for those with hypertension of panic disorder. The alternative practice in this case is Ujjayi Breath…

To begin, as we always do, get into a comfortable sitting position, and begin to relax by breathing deep and long, extending your exhalations to increase the relaxation messages to the body and mind.

When ready, inhale to 70/80% of your lung capacity, pause, and then exhale through the nose forcefully, as if you are sneezing. You will feel your abdomen engaging and your navel moving towards your spine. Repeat a few times to help your body get used to the feeling. You may feel a little lightheaded, but this is normal and nothing to worry about.

When you are ready, start your practice with 10 forceful exhalations through the nostrils, and then slowly exhale completely. Each cycle should be one second and the tempo should be even. Inhale deeply and exhale completely twice and on the 3rd inhale, hold your breath. Close your eyes and focus and the area between your eyebrows or the area at your heart centre. Hold your breath for as long as you are comfortable. The main aim is not to stress the body in any way and remember this is not a competition and there is no benefit to holding your breath for an extended period if it stresses the lungs and body. If there is any breathlessness, then the breath has been held for too long.

Now, repeat the process two more times, the second time with 12 exhalations and the third time with 15 exhalations. Over time, advance your practice and increase the forceful exhalations, always keeping in mind that the most benefit from this exercise is attained by working within your capacity and never being breathless. Try not to put the cart before the horse. Keep in mind that advanced practitioners generally do three rounds of 120, 130 and finish with 150 pumps.

What is the Science?

During the practice of Kapalabhatti, the levels of Carbon Dioxide (CO_2) in the blood substantially drop quickly. Although this is abnormal, it is beneficial to the body. The normal level of CO_2 is re-established soon after the end of the practice. So, is there any point in doing this exercise? What is the actual benefit? This temporary drop in CO_2 in the blood give the cells a chance to eliminate their own CO_2. As this happens, the cells become saturated with Oxygen and this activity is very important for the general population who live a mostly sedentary life. This cellular respiration harvests energy in the body for immediate or later use.

Along with purifying the lungs and maintaining it suppleness, the exercise maintains the mobility of the diaphragm and strengthens the abdominal muscles.

Along with all this, it is a tonic for the whole nervous system. After a long stressful day, it is the ideal practice to recover lost vitality. Use it to regain freshness, clear the mind of that muddled feeling and banish any hint of lethargy and listlessness. Watch how regular practice will help you with your concentration levels and improves your memory.

15. Bhastrika – The Bellows Breath

If you have ever used a bellows or seen one in operation, you will notice that the outflow of air is much more powerful than the inflow. The inflow is gentle and subtle, and the outflow is forceful and sudden. This is the picture you will have in your mind and the feeling you will have in your body as you perform this practice. The importance of slowly introducing Bhastrika into your practice cannot be stressed enough. As it is a forceful practice, it can put stress on your lungs, abdomen and heart and should be introduced slowly and calmly.

Sitting in a comfortable position, arms straight, hands resting on legs or knees, palms facing down, fingers wide apart. Practice your three-part breath for a few breaths and release tension from your body each time you exhale.

To begin, as you inhale, raise both arms above your head, elbows into your ears and fingers wide apart. Picture the bellows and the gentle, subtle inflow of air.

After a very slight pause at the top of the breath, close your fingers and make a tight fist with both hands. Keep the picture of the bellows in your mind. Exhale forcefully and quickly, bringing your elbows down quickly to the sides of your ribs. Now, straighten your arms again, placing them back on your legs, knees, opening your hands and fingers and repeat the process.

For beginners, this should be repeated three to five times, as appropriate. This will be one round. At the end of a round (3-5 forced exhalations), inhale to 70/80% of your lung capacity and hold your breath until you feel that you need to breathe again. There is no record to be broken here for breath retention, just listen to your body and react to its signals. Repeat for three rounds and remember, at no time should the body be put under stress, ever. This is a very powerful practice and should not be practiced first in a breathwork routine. The body should be prepared, with Kapalabhatti generally. As these are hyperventilation practices, care should be taken. Gradual progression is the key to success and eventually reaching twenty pumps per round is sufficient to attain the maximum benefits of the practice.

The science behind the practice is the same as Kapalabhatti and helps with our energy levels and focus.

16. Lose Weight!..Just Breathe!

According to researchers from the University of New South Wales in Australia, when weight is lost, most of it is breathed out as carbon dioxide. The study was originally published in the British Medical Journal in December 2014 by Ruben Meerman and Andrew Brown. Ruben Meerman also wrote a book on the subject, Big Fat Myths. This was a little like re-inventing the wheel as this basic information was built on the discovery by the French scientist, Antoine Lavoisier in the late 1700s. The basic theory is that Food + Oxygen is transformed to Carbon Dioxide and Water (Food + O2 = CO2 + H2O). Respiration/Breathing is combustion.

They discovered that there was widespread confusion about how weight is lost. Most of us believe that it is sweated out of our bodied, excreted within faeces or converted to muscle.

The results of this new and old research suggest and then goes on to prove that the lungs are the main excretory organ for weight loss, with the H_2O produced by oxidation departing the body in urine, faeces, breath, and other bodily fluids. From this information and the above equation, we see that the rest of the weight loss comes from CO2 (Carbon Dioxide) in our Exhalations. In fact, and surprisingly, for every 10kg of body weight that we lose, 8.4Kg is lost through exhalation. I noticed that the first time I gave this statistic at a conference, the whole room suddenly sat bolt upright in their chairs. This was big news! They were hooked! It is well worth repeating. Eighty Four Percent of lost weight is breathed out of your body.

Even those of us with a basic science education can appreciate that if we inhale O2 (2 Atoms) and we exhale CO2 (3 Atoms), our exhalation is heavier than our inhalation. For a practical example from Meerman; If we eat a large Burger and Fries, it will take 13 hours to exhale the Carbon Dioxide produced if we stay inactive. If we walk, it will take over 6 hours and if we go for a jog, it will take just over 3 hours.

The Carbon Dioxide that is lost through exhalation/exercise is only replaced through the consumption of food and beverages. Keeping our body weight stable or decreasing it simply requires that we put less back into our bodies by eating less than we have exhaled by breathing. Extending our exhalations slowly, using Pranayama techniques, a little less eating and a little more moving, brings us to a place where we can exert control over our weight.

The line from the Meerman and Brown study sums up all of this information very simply:

"Lungs are therefore the primary excretory organ for weight loss"

17. Nadi Shodhana – Alternate Nostril Breathing

I must admit that when the difference between breathing through my left and right nostril was revealed to me in India, I became a little obsessed with the process. Even now, when I wake in the morning, I check to see which nostril I am breathing through and I then always place the same foot on the floor first. So, left nostril, left foot, right nostril, right foot. Start the day on the right foot! Of course, it also tells me what tasks I should start the day with. There is no point in starting the day with a logical task, left brain activity, if I wake up with a dominant left nostril. If my right brain is active, then my day should start with some reading of fiction, maybe sing along to some uplifting music, or write some imaginative piece. All these right brain activities flourish when your breathing is dominant in your left nostril. Paying your bills and dealing with your finances is a good early morning activity when you wake you with a dominant right nostril and a logical mindset. Perish the thought. The left nostril is a cooling breath and connected to the lunar while and the right nostril is a warming breath and connect to the solar.

To begin, sit in a comfortable position, spine straight. As always, before beginning any practice, inhale deeply and exhale completely through your nostrils, bringing the body and mind into a relaxed state.

Place your left hand in Chin/Jnana Mudra, resting on your knee or leg. This applies to both left and right-handed practitioners. Now, we will introduce a fourth mudra. Place your right thumb on your right nostril, gently closing the nostril. Fold your index and middle finger into your palm and keep your little finger and ring finger straight. This is Vishnu Mudra. Check that your chin is parallel to the floor.

With the right nostril closed, inhale for 3-4 seconds through the left nostril – Om1, Om2, Om3, Om4 – rotate your wrist so that your little finger and ring finger close the left nostril, release your thumb from your right nostril and exhale through the right nostril, Om1, Om2, Om3, Om4. Now, inhale on the right for a count of four, close the right nostril with your thumb, release the little and ring finger, and exhale through the left nostril for a count of four. This is one round. If a count of four is too much for either the inhale of the exhale, then reduce to a count of three and begin your practice from there. It is important to equalise the ratio of your breathing to begin with. Slowly increase the length of inhale and exhale to the limit that is within your ability. Any breathlessness, light-headedness or forcing of the breath is too extreme. Take a step back and listen to your body. Focus on the area between your eyebrows of your heart centre. Over time, the need to count will diminish as you will be aware of the limits of your body and a natural rhythm will establish itself.

This is the beginning of your practice. To progress, it is important that the exhalation is extended for a longer period than the inhalation, and so the equal 1:1 ratio will change. As with all breathing exercises, steady progress is the aim. Eventually reaching a 1:2 ratio is the goal for this exercise. So, inhaling for 3, exhaling for 6, and so on up. Four, eight is a nice rhythm, and inhale for a count of eight is the highest one should practice.

What are the benefits of this simple practice to our bodies and minds?

- Infuses the body with oxygen
- Clears and releases toxins
- Reduces stress and anxiety
- Calms and rejuvenates the nervous system
- Clear and balances the respiratory channels
- Helps to alleviate respiratory allergies
- Balances solar and lunar energy
- Improves mental clarity and an alert mind
- Enhances the ability to concentrate
- Brings balance to the left and right hemispheres of the brain

18. Anuloma Viloma – Alternate Nostril Breathing w/ Breath Retention.

Having become comfortable with Nadi Shodhana, you can now progress to Anuloma Viloma. The simple difference between each practice is that the breath is retained between inhalation and exhalation. Pinch the nostrils to stop the breath, relax, and retain.

To begin, return to the 1:1:1 ratio. Sitting in your comfortable position, inhale through your left nostril for a count of 4, retain your breath, by pinching your nostrils for a count of 4, release your thumb and exhale for a count of 4 through your right nostril. Now, inhale through right nostril for 4, retain breath for a count of 4 and then exhale through left nostril for a count of 4. This is one round. It is important to practice this rhythm until you are relaxed and comfortable throughout the process.

What does progress in this practice look like? How will you change the ratio to reach the first goal of Anuloma Viloma? What is the ratio goal to aim for?

Begin with slowly increasing the length of the breath retention and exhalation. Get comfortable with the feeling and the change of ratio. To begin with, there is no need to count. Just let your body and mind be comfortable with the extensions. Inhale for the count of four – left nostril, hold your breath, relax, exhale through right nostril, and continue.

As you and your body and mind become comfortable in the practice, you can now begin to focus on the ratio. For this practice, the final exhalation should be twice the length of the inhalation e.g. inhale for four, exhale for eight. The aim is to reach the ratio 1:4:2, so a count of four, sixteen, eight. Again, steady progress to this goal is what is needed. Never retain your breath beyond the limit of your capacity and build slowly, steadily, and comfortably. If you decide to test yourself, long-term, the maximum inhale should not exceed a count of eight and best of luck!

We have already seen the benefits of Nadi Shodhana, and these also apply to Anuloma Viloma, but added to this because of the breath

retention and increased CO2 in the blood, the following can also be added to the benefits:
- Elevated carbon dioxide promotes healing of lung tissues.
- Regulates the blood Ph levels
- Relaxes muscle cells and releases tension
- Haemoglobin proteins release their oxygen

19.Surya and Chandra Bheda – The Sun, Moon

As mentioned earlier, the nostrils are a gateway to better health. As well as serving us as our inbuilt air-conditioning system, they also balance the flow of oxygen to the left and right side of the brain.

The left nostril cools and is connected to the coolness of the

Moon (Chandra) and the right nostril is connected the heat and warmth of the Sun (Surya). Because our nostrils can be used to bring about physiological changes, we can use breathing techniques to take advantage of these characteristics. Interestingly the idea of hot and cold can also be associated with mood and these practices can be used in this are also. We have all heard the term and have described people or ourselves as, "hot under the collar" and also "cold as ice" to describe being angry or excited over something or being unattached or removed from a situation or person, respectively . When we are angry or excited, we need to cool down and when we are removed/unattached we need to connect or be warmer.

Sometimes we need to focus on a project or a task at hand. We need to fire up and stimulate our left brain. At other times we need to fire up our creativity and visualisation.

So, cool or heat your body, change your mood, and stimulate your brain in a simple breathing technique.

Sitting in your favoured position, close your right nostril with your right thumb and inhale through your left nostril (Moon, Cooling, Right Brain Oxygenation). Rotate wrist and close left nostril with little and ring finger. Exhale through right nostril. Close right nostril with thumb when exhale completed. This is one round. Inhale through left nostril again and continue for at least five rounds. To advance the practice, hold your breath comfortably after inhalation and extend exhalation to empty lungs. There is no need for ratio breathing in this exercise. Just proceed in a stress-free manner.

Closing your left nostril with your little and ring finger and inhaling through your right nostril (Sun, Heating, Left Brain Oxygenation), continue with the practice, inhaling only through the right nostril and exhaling only through the left nostril.

It is advised to **practice only one** of the above on any given day.

Surya Bheda Pranayama activates the body and the bodily functions. It increases the digestive fire. It destroys all diseases that are caused by insufficiency of oxygen in the blood. The ancient yoga text, The Gheranda Samhita says that Surya Bheda Pranayama destroys decay and death, awakens Kundalini Shakti, and increases digestive fire.

Chandra Bheda reduces body heat and relieves heart burn. It refreshes the body and mind and reduces blood pressure. It is also useful to practice when trying to reduce fever in the body

20. Sitali and Sitkari Pranayama – Cooling/Hissing Breath

For those of you who live in a climate where there can be hot and humid weather, these practices can be a great help to relieve the overwhelming feeling that this type of weather can induce. I have been told that these techniques are generally only used during the Monsoon season. Practicing in a temperate or cool environment can lead to a sore throat and even bronchial issues. As you will see, they involve breathing with an open mouth, so they are used only for a specific situation.

After taking a few deep long and slow breaths, form an "O" with your lips, pointing and folding your tongue into the space. Wait for saliva to form on the tongue and take a slow, long, inhale, letting the air slowly pass over the tongue. When you finish inhaling, close your lips, and slowly exhale through your nose. Practice for between 3-5 minutes.

Some of us are not genetically predisposed to make this rolled shape with our tongues and practice Sitali. If this is the case, then you can practice

Sitkari/Hissing Breath. It is the same practice but with a variation in the tongue position.

Press your teeth together, open your lips and expose your teeth. Fold your tongue, so that the underside is pressed up into the roof of your mouth. Slowly inhale and draw in the moistened air through the sides of your mouth. When finished, close your mouth and exhale slowly and completely.

Benefits listed for this practice are:

- Cooling the entire body, nervous system, and brain.
- Helps deal with stress, anger, and anxiety.
- Therapeutic for insomnia.
- Lowers the Blood Pressure.

21. Just say NO!..The joys of Nitric Oxide

Nitric Oxide is a molecule that is produced naturally by your body. It is important for many aspects of your health. Its most important function is to relax the inner muscles of the blood vessels, causing them to widen and increase circulation. This is called vasodilation.

Nitric oxide production is essential for overall health because it allows blood, nutrients, and oxygen to travel to every part of your body effectively and efficiently.

In fact, a limited capacity to produce nitric oxide is associated with heart disease, diabetes, and erectile dysfunction.

Fortunately, there are many ways to maintain optimal levels of nitric oxide in your body. The most effective method is nasal breathing and to boost production exponentially, just hum while inhaling and exhaling through your nose. The practice of Brahmari Breathing is essential for this. Before moving on to this let us take a quick look at other ways.

Here are the top ways to increase nitric oxide naturally.

When you eat food that is high in Nitrates, this is converted to Nitric Oxide in the body. These foods include, Celery, Beetroot, Spinach and Lettuce. A recent study by the University of Exeter found that athletes who drank beetroot juice (480ml/1 Pint per day for 7 days) showed a huge reduction in the amount of oxygen required to perform exercise. The numbers were impressive with a 16% increase in endurance for cyclists. Coupled with a reduction in blood pressure, they concluded that this reduction in the need for oxygen to increase endurance could not be achieved by any other training method.

Nitric oxide is an unstable molecule that degrades quickly in the bloodstream, so it must be constantly replenished. One way to increase its stability and limit its breakdown and degradation is by consuming antioxidants.

Antioxidants are molecules that neutralize free radicals, which contribute to the short life of nitric oxide. These antioxidants are found in all foods but primarily those of plant origin, such as fruits, vegetables, nuts, seeds, and grains. Increasing our intake of Vitamin C and E are the easiest way to increase antioxidants in the body.

Avoid mouthwash. Mouthwash kills many types of bacteria including the ones that produce nitric oxide. This limits the ability of your body to produce Nitric Oxide.

Finally, have a long-term, steady, exercise routine. Because we are discussing Pranayama and the control of breath, the word steady is important here. Let us add the word comfortable too. Most importantly, while exercising, keep your mouth closed and only inhale and exhale through your nose. For those who are generally mouth breathers, this will seem strange and you may find yourself struggling to breath. Do not quit. Keep your focus. Begin your practice and new health habit while walking and build towards more exertive exercise, running, rowing, hiking etc. It will not take long to get comfortable, but the benefit will outweigh any initial discomfort. One aspect of exercise that tends to be overlooked is exercising and strengthening the Diaphragm, our main breathing muscle.

22. Black Bee Breath – Brahmari

Sitting on a rooftop at dawn, eyes closed, focusing on the area between them, listening to the frogs loudly greeting a new day from the rice paddies below is a unique experience. Add to this the sound of a swarm of female black bees and it can be a little disconcerting, to say the least. Everybody in our group is humming, the sounds melt together and the air fills and vibrates with the sound. It feels as if the group exhalation lasts for 10 minutes uninterrupted. The vibration of the sound is on all our lips, but the feeling moves throughout the body and especially resonates in the spinal column.

This is where I first learned Brahmari – The Black Bee Breath and I have been hooked ever since. It is said that when an advanced Yogi practices this technique, supreme bliss is attained. Coupled with this promise, it is the most efficient method of naturally producing Nitric Oxide in the sinuses, the benefits of which we have already seen. While humming can be used as an introduction to this technique and can also produce Nitric Oxide (NO), Brahmari breathing turbo charges the production but also calms the body and mind. The health benefits of Nitric Oxide are being realised through recent scientific research as we will see later.

It is advised that this technique should only be practiced by those who are adept at slow and deep breathing.

Sitting with a straight spine, inhaling through the nose, very slightly restrict the passage of air between the nasal passage and the throat. You will feel your lips and mouth vibrate. The sound is described as that of a drone bee. The inhalation may seem short and difficult to extend, this is normal. The exhalation is of greater significance in this practice and so it is named after the sound of the exhalation. When exhaling, again having slightly restricted the breath between the throat and the nasal passage, slowly exhale, and remove all the breath from your lungs. Do not strain to make the sound last. It should fade away as if the bee is fading out of earshot, not stopping, just fading. This is an ideal practice to time and I generally do 3-5 minutes. Of course, it can also be done with several breaths, 5/10/20 etc. For such a simple calm practice, the physical benefits are enormous.

To begin, the sound of the inhalation and exhalation may be a little jumpy with slight gaps, but this will improve and become continuous and unbroken.

To bring your awareness inward and rest in the vibration of the black bee, lightly place a finger in both ears while exhaling.

The benefits of Brahmari are listed as:

- It increases the production on Nitric Oxide in the nasal passage
- It assists in the reduction of stress. ...
- It lowers blood pressure, thus relieving hypertension.
- It releases cerebral tension.
- It soothes the nerves.
- It stimulates the pineal and pituitary glands, thus supporting their proper functioning.
- It dissipates anger.
- It is helpful in preventing heart blockages
- It helps with inducing deep sleep

23.Other Breathing Methods……

Buteko was developed by Konstantin Buteyko, a Ukrainian doctor in the 1950's. He discovered that over breathing or hyperventilation was the root of many diseases, especially diseases of the respiratory system such as asthma. The Buteko method is said to help with many illnesses including, hay fever, sleep apnoea, snoring, high blood pressure, anxiety, and low energy levels.

Tummo, which literally means 'inner fire', is an ancient meditation technique practiced by monks in Tibetan Buddhism. Tummo exists of a combination of breathing and visualization techniques, used to enter a deep state of meditation that is used to increase a person's 'inner heat'.

Wim Hof, Dutch extreme athlete Wim Hof got his nickname "The Iceman" by breaking a number of records related to cold exposure including: climbing Mount Kilimanjaro in shorts, running a half marathon above the Arctic Circle barefoot, and standing in a container while covered with ice cubes for more than 112 minutes.

Using "cold, hard nature" as his teacher, his extensive training has enabled him to learn to control his breathing, heart rate, and blood circulation and to withstand extreme temperatures. A 2014 study injecting Wim Hof Method practitioners with an endotoxin, showed they were able to control their sympathetic nervous system and immune response. This could mean that the Wim Hof Method is an effective tool to battle symptoms of various autoimmune diseases.

Holotrophic:

This breathing technique is generally practiced in a group setting. Participants are paired as a "breather" and a "sitter". The breathing involves rapid deep inhaling and exhaling in a rhythm to avoid hyperventilation, the purpose of which is to obtain enlightenment of some kind.

Proponents of this technique contend that this altered state allows people to access parts of the mind that are not usually accessible; this might include memories of past events and traumas.

Somatic:

This method of breathing therapy can be done either sitting up or lying down on the back. The breath is intentionally engaged with no pauses between inhale and exhale. The breath can flow either in and out of the nose or mouth. By breathing this way your body naturally begins to release physical tension and surface levels of stress. As you learn to breathe diaphragmatically, this type of breathing has the capacity to release deeper emotional and mental patterns.

Sudharsan Kriya:

This breathing technique is promoted by the Art of Living organisation, founded by Sri Sri Ravi Shankar 'Su' means proper, and 'darshan' means vision. 'Kriya' in yogic science means to purify the body. Sudarshan Kriya means 'proper vision by purifying action.' Sudarshan Kriya involves cyclical breathing patterns that range from slow and calming to rapid and stimulating. In this Kriya, you take control of your breath, which positively affects your immune system, nerves, and psychological problems.

According to a 2009 published study of Harvard Medical School, Sudarshan Kriya yoga can effectively address anxiety and depression.

DeRose Method

This breathing method is promoted by the Brazilian yoga teacher, Luiz DeRose. Based on Yogic Pranayama techniques.

Hypoventilation

Hypoventilation is a physical training method in which periods of exercise with reduced breathing frequency are interspersed with periods with normal breathing. The hypoventilation technique consists of short breath holdings and can be performed in different types of exercise: running, cycling etc.

Generally, there are two ways to carry out hypoventilation: they involve holding the breath at full lung volume and at low lung volume.

Breath Holding

In general, basic breath holding while exercising can lead to increased fitness and improved endurance. Multiple studies have shown that using this basic method of breathwork has improved the performance of athletes and is a valid substitute for high altitude training. Although there are benefits from holding the breath in the body, the benefits are increased by exhaling and holding the breath outside the body. The ideal exercise for this is Samma Vritti. It takes time to implement this into exercise, but try to introduce slowly while walking and then add to other exercise routines, jogging, running, cycling etc.

24. Relax like a Corpse – Play Dead

In a Yoga practice, we relax, before and after our postures. We know this as Shavasana (Corpse Pose). It is regarded, on the one hand, as the most difficult pose, and on the other hand, as the most important pose, in a student's practice. Both viewpoints are true. It is also an important practice after Pranayama as it assists the body in assimilating the energy created by the practice. It is easy to imagine our energy being blocked by tension in any area of our bodies and so to increase the flow of this fresh energy (Prana), we need to give time over to relaxation. How do we achieve this?

For some students, because of agility issues, it is not possible to lie on the floor for Shavasana. This is not an issue. They can just stay seated on a chair, spine straight, not supported by the back of the chair and go through the process. For others, lie down on a Yoga mat or a blanket on the floor. Feet out to the corners of the mat/blanket, hands away from the body, palms facing up. Take a few deep long breaths…. mouth closed!

Full relaxation is achieved by autosuggestion. So, to begin, tense and relax different parts of your body systematically. Tense and relax the legs, the abdomen, chest, arms, face, and any other areas that work for you. Do this slowly.

Next, systematically relax each separate part of your body, both externally and internally. Start with your toes, and repeat to yourself, "relax my toes" and do this for each body part as you move upward towards the head and face.

Relax my feet, relax my ankles, relax my calf muscles, shins, thighs, hips, back, spine, abdomen, internal organs (name as many as you can), fingers, hands, arms, shoulders, neck, head, face, mouth, tongue and finish with the chin.

Now, the energy can flow freely throughout the body with no blocks and we can experience the full benefits of the breathing exercises. Take as much time as you can to do this. Even three to five minutes is good, but ten minutes is better. It can also be a good idea to set an alarm while doing this, as the body can fall into a deep sleep. When finished, slowly roll to your right-hand side, take a couple of breaths, slowly sit up, and then stand up.

Now, you have filled each part of your body with new and fresh energy. Remember that both physical and emotional actions and reactions will feed off this energy, so use it wisely.

25.Conclusion

I have written this book as an introduction to Pranayama and Breathwork and to introduce the reader to the health benefits of proper breathing. Again, the word "simple" in the title is there for a purpose. I have tried to simplify the techniques, the science and theory. I hope that it is accessible to the vast majority of people and can be of benefit to everyone. Take the time to just practice a little of what is written here.

There are many fads and fashions in our world today, but these ancient practices have been handed down to us and have stood the test of time. They are easy to learn and can be inserted into our daily life and routines with ease. How difficult is it to practice while sitting in traffic, the subway, bus, or train? How difficult is it to just close your mouth and focus on the feeling of the breath in your nostrils? The cool air on the inhale and the warm air on the exhale. The calmness of the mind.

Breathe Deeper, Breathe Longer, Breathe Slower, Breathe Less.

Close your Mouth.

Let us finish with the Sanskrit Proverb,

"For breath is life, so if you breathe well, you will live long on this earth"

NAMASTE

Dermot Ryan

After many years of travel in India I began my Yoga journey in 2013.

Having completed my Teacher Training Certification in 2016 at the Aarsha Yoga Vidya Peetham in India I then completed my Advanced Teacher Training Certification (RYT 500) in February 2018 at the Sivananda Yoga Vidya Peetham under the guidance of the renowned teacher Swami Govindananda Saraswati

I practice and teach Yoga in the traditional way as taught in the Sivananda Yoga Tradition. The five points of the tradition are, Proper Exercise, Proper Breathing, Proper Relaxation, Proper Diet and Positive Thinking/Meditation.

OM Purnamadah Purnamidam Purnat Purnamudachyate

Purnasya Purnamadaya Purnamevavashisyate

OM, Shantih, Shantih, Shantih

Printed in Great Britain
by Amazon